THE POWER OF

POSITIVE PARENTING

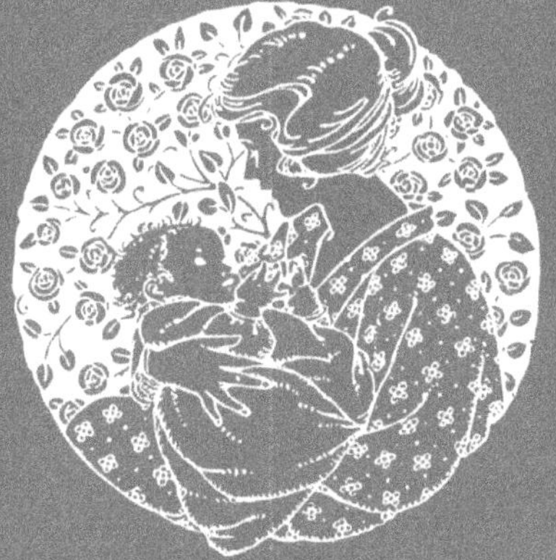

Francis .A. Uwandu

THE POWER OF POSITIVE PARENTING

BY

FRANCIS A. UWANDU

©2023

DEDICATION

I dedicate this book to my mum, Late Mrs. Augusta Uwandu for her unflinching love, courage and support towards me and my siblings. She was indeed a super woman and my very own superhero. Thank you mum for all you went through just to see us become what you desired us to be. You deserve this and much more.

INTRODUCTION

The rate at which the spirit of disobedience has crept into the heart and minds of children in this generation is alarming.

Children are being manipulated every day to do evil and ungodly things.

Just the other day, a seven year old girl was rushed to the hospital for virginal bleeding. After a brief interrogation it was found out that her class mate injected a sharp object into her virgina. When the young lad who injected the object into her was asked how he came about such an evil act, he responded that their house help taught him. He had seen her injecting a sexual stimulant into her virgina and he decided to try it on his classmate.

A teenager was caught by his parents masturbating. He was hitting his penis against the wall. When they got to the doctor, they realized that he had damaged his manhood. The continuous friction on the wall had affected his erection.

I can go on and on to tell you of the alarming every day occurrences happening in the world of the adolescent and the teenager.

It is glaring that parents need to take responsibility in the upbringing of their children. We shouldn't leave all the work for their teachers, house helps, and guardians.

Parents have a stronger bond with their children. God has given us the core responsibility of child upbringing. We have to train our children in a way and manner that God will be pleased.

This book has been carefully written with powerful insights to help you secure the destiny and future of your children. Their tomorrow begins today.

Read through and get divine wisdom to help you give your children the best for the benefit of their future.

Chapter 1

Know Your Child

Proverbs 29:15 The rod and reproof give wisdom: but a child left to himself bringeth his mother to shame.

Dear parents, it is on a sad note I am writing to you.

As parents, our busy schedules have deprived us of taking responsibility to foster our children. We leave for work very early and return home very late. We leave for work when our children are still asleep and return when they are fast asleep. And even when we are at home on weekends, we barely spend quality time with them. We would rather hang out with friends or go watch football when we are supposed to get to know our children better.

When the school calls for Parents Teachers Association meetings, we are too busy to attend. We rather send their nanny or our maid to cover up for us. And when something goes wrong, we blame every other person except ourselves. This is how cold, self centered, hard heartened, and careless we have become.

In the formative years of childhood, children are to be bonded by their parents. Parents are to be very close to their children. That early stage of upbringing is very vital for the baby.

Behaviors like breast feeding and bathing the baby creates a special bond between baby and mother.

When we had our first baby, it came to a point where I had to begin to bathe the baby. I didn't want to do it at first. But I wanted to have a bond with my baby so this made me do it. Those touches on her tender skin brings a bond between parents and children that are special.

When we have a special bond with our children, it becomes easy to train them. But when we don't do this, it becomes difficult to create that attachment that will last a lifetime and this can have a negative impact on our children. And if any misfortune befalls them, we will be held accountable.

God kept them in our care and not in the care of the house help, the nanny, the pastor, the Sunday school teacher, and (or) the class teacher.

But I must warn us here, kindly ensure to have equal emotional attachment with your children. It's dangerous to love one more than the other or be too emotionally attached to one than the other. This behavior can crumble your home and cause an everlasting hatred between siblings.

We saw how Rebecca, Isaac's wife, almost destroyed her home by showing more affection for one child than the other. This brought discord between brothers and created a separation that it took God to fix after a long period of time.

We also saw this behavior repeating itself in the life of Jacob. His mother chose him over his brother. And we saw him being emotionally attached with Rachael's children more than the children of the other women. And this brought trouble to the one who receives more of his attention than the others. His love for Joseph over his brothers made them hate him and almost killed him. It also brought Jacob pain. The pain of losing a beloved son.

So learn to love your children evenly. Teach them how to love one another and be there for each other. Preach the gospel of togetherness among your children. Make no mistake of putting one child over the other or comparing one child to another. Make no mistake of capitalizing on the strength of one child over the weakness of the other. Remember that your children have their own individual uniqueness. Don't set your home ablaze with the fires of hatred, jealousy, envy, and distrust.

Don't give room for unhealthy comparisons. It's not worth it.

2 Samuel 4:4

And Jonathan, Saul's son, had a son that was lame of his feet. He was five years old when the tidings came of Saul and Jonathan out of Jezreel, and his nurse took him up, and fled: and it came to pass, as she made haste to flee, that he fell, and became lame. And his name was Mephibosheth.

From the above verse, we can see how this little child accidentally fell off from the nurse and injured his feet which made him crippled for life. Would he have fallen if it was his mother that carried him? She would be careful not to make him slip off her hands.

This is one of the dangers amidst others of having someone else take care of our child or children when we are too busy.

Proverbs 29:15 says, '....but a child left to himself disgraces his mother'. What does this mean? It means that if you do not take time to know your child/children and correct them when they go astray, they will bring you shame and reproach when you least expect it.

Ephesians 6:4

And, ye fathers, provoke not your children to wrath: but bring them up in the nurture and admonition of the Lord.

The above verse did not say, 'Pastor, Sunday school teacher, class teacher, or lesson teacher. It says, 'Fathers.'

As fathers it is our utmost responsibility to train up our child/children in the way of the Lord. To achieve this, we must take responsibility and quit shifting all the work to our wives, and (or) our mothers. We must take sole responsibility to the upbringing of our child(ren).

We must make out time and reschedule our plans to fit into God's plan for our children. We are the architect of whatever happens in our home.

The role of the father in the upbringing of a child is very important. Mothers also have a good role to play but both are unique and the combination of the both makes the training impactful.

The absence of a father affects the child both now and in the future. Things tend to go wrong when the father is never around.

A father guards the gate of the house from strangers and enemies that want to penetrate his home and destroy his family. He watches in prayer and safeguards the entire household. Mummy and the children feel safe and secure when daddy is around. He is the one in charge and in authority as the head of his household.

They are things mummy cannot handle because she is not empowered in that area. When the enemy of your household realizes that daddy is not always around, he will look for a way to come into the house and make a mess of it before daddy returns.

This was what happened with Adam and Eve. The devil took advantage of Adam's absence to deceive his wife and mess up the home before he returned.

As fathers, our eyes must remain on our family. We must watch over them and cover them in prayers no matter how far we are. Sometimes fathers have to travel long distances and spend days or weeks on an assignment before returning home. When this happens, we must watch over them with prayers, and phone calls. We must ask God to keep them from evil and keep evil far from them and your entire household.

God's angels can protect your family on your behalf, even in your absence if you pray. Your household can remain in one piece if you engage God's angels prayerfully no matter where you are. This you must do as a father to keep your entire family safe and secure.

Family Comes First

Family is more important than anything else. A lot of us parents make the mistake of putting our jobs, businesses, ministries, and other things as first priority before the love and commitment we have to show to our family.

A wife who is a banker should first consider the well-being of her family before considering the well-being of the bank.

We must understand that our family is the closest to us. Any job or business whose intent is to take you far away from your loved ones should be reconsidered and carefully thought through. We cannot allow our jobs to deprive us of the responsibility of taking proper care of our family.

For it is disastrous to leave the flinty fire on the roof of our house burning and focus on quenching the little flames of fire on another person's roof.

A lot of families have been destroyed and a lot of homes have become a war zone because of negligence on the part of the parents in the family.

Family is the first ministry given to us by God. The devil knows the importance of a united home so he does all he can to scatter the foundations in families.

Everyone first belongs to a home before belonging to a society. If love, peace, tender kindness and togetherness are exhibited in the home, it will reflect in the society.

All the evil committed by man in society is as a result of broken homes. Those who became rebels, terrorists, armed robbers, rapists, ritual killers, serial killers, drug Lords, kingpins, prostitutes and so on grew up from a home. Their parents neglected the core aspect of training up their children and they became wasted youths over the years.

Nobody was born a thief, a felon, an armed robber, or a prostitute. Humans naturally gravitate to where they are loved, cared for, cherished, and celebrated. The heat and hatred at home may drive, propel or move one to where they could find a little bit of love and care, and even if they found love in the wrong place, that place eventually becomes their home. They become a duplicate of the product in the environment they find themselves in.

In the bible, Samuel and Eli's children were the direct opposite of their fathers. They lived wayward lives which were contrary to the life their fathers lived. This may be as a result of negligence in the upbringing of their sons. They were probably too busy doing God's work and thereby not having quality time to take care of things in their household.

We should not be too busy doing other people's work while we leave ours undone. Even as men of God. We need to apply wisdom and attend to the immediate needs of our family.

1 Timothy 3:1 This is a true saying, If a man desires the office of a bishop, he desireth a good work.

1 Timothy 3:4-5

One that ruled his own house, having his children in subjection with all gravity; (For if a man knows not how to rule his own house, how shall he take care of the church of God?.

From the above we can see how serious God takes the appropriateness of taking good care of the family. As a minister of the gospel of Jesus Christ, the devil's number one target is your family. He wants to get back at you for all the damages you are doing to his kingdom. He wants people to point accusing fingers on your children and utter hurting, and hateful words at you.

This is why we must be sensitive, sober, and vigilant as regards issues pertaining to our home. Don't leave your wife to do all the training. Women weren't mentioned in the above Bible verse as core trainers to the raising of a child. You have to protect your family and keep demons completely off them. So you and them do not become a laughing stock at the end of the day.

I was asking God to give me good children. He replied saying, 'All the children I give to men are good. They only have to bring them up in the way of the Lord.'

Ephesians 6:4

And, ye fathers, provoke not your children to wrath: but bring them up in the nurture and admonition of the Lord.

If you're having a family dispute right now, stop laying the blame on your wife. Look where you have failed in your responsibility to bring up your child(ren) in the way and admonition of the Lord. Accept corrections and ask God for mercy and forgiveness. God will then accept your request and enable you with divine wisdom to build your home in a way and manner that pleases him.

He will give you the wisdom to manage both his work and your home, thereby becoming a success both in your family upbringing and in your ministry.

Chapter 2

Mind What You Do Oh Man!

Be careful what you do around your children. They do what they see you do. As children grow up, they naturally practice what they see at home, at school, in church and in every place they find themselves. You have to be careful to watch them and rebuke them when they exhibit characters that are ungodly. It is a huge task but you have to create time to build them up so that you don't cry over them tomorrow.

Children replicate what they see their parents do. In fact, they do what they see on television and sing out the pieces of music they hear at home and when they go out.

A man came to my mum back then to complain to her about her son who smokes. When he left our house, she told us how a terrible smoker the man was. His son would have of course learnt this from his dad.

You shouldn't begin to blame your children when they go the wrong way, especially when it is exactly what you do. They have picked it from you so judging them also brings you into judgment.

Romans 2:1 Therefore thou art inexcusable, O man, whosoever thou art that judgest: for wherein thou judgest another, thou condemnest thyself; for thou that judgest does the same things.

Your child is a product of you. It is what they see you do they will do. Don't be surprised when you see them do good or ugly things the way you do them. If you want to see them do things differently, do things differently.

As a parent, it is within your power to control what your children watch on television or listen to on the radio. It's within your power to control the kind of games they play and the kind of places they go.

If you buy any educational or entertaining resource from the market, please watch them first. If you find anything that will negatively influence their communication, emotions and actions, avoid introducing the materials to them. Do not say, "I can't just allow my money to go to waste so they have to watch it that way." if you can take it back and exchange it for another please do. If you can't, kindly get rid of it. It is better your money go to waste than allowing that material to destroy the lives of your children.

When you fail to put parental control on the channels of your decoder, you are exposing your children to unfriendly influences capable of destroying their character formation.

It is your duty to make out time and observe the different channels on the decoder and control the ones they can watch. If that seems to be like a huge task to accomplish, you can only subscribe to channels that will positively help their upbringing.

If you also think the above is not a good option, you can get two decoders, one for you and your wife and the other for your kids. You can only subscribe to educational and entertaining channels for them and as they grow into the adolescents and teenagers you desire, you can add more milder channels to help develop other aspects of their minds.

If you also think this might be expensive, then go for decoders which have channels that have more religious and educational materials. This will equally help your children's mental health as you watch them grow. Don't be of the opinion that they can watch anything. If you allow this line of thought to set in, your children will bring disgrace to you and you will be badly affected by this.

The media is full of dirty things that can corrupt the innocent minds of little children. So be careful to filter your mobile phones before handing them over to your kids. Some dirty videos may automatically download into your phone through Whatsapp or through any other mobile application on your mobile device or gadget.

You may not be aware that a new video has automatically been downloaded into your phone gallery. But if you always check your phone properly before they do, this can help you do a thorough check on your mobile device before handing it over to them.

It's also advisable that you put a password on your phone and do a routine check always before handing it over to them. This is very important.

If they have access to a laptop, kindly check their browsing history to see if they haven't been introduced to sites that can mess up their minds so that they don't begin to do ugly things in private while everyone is asleep.

Children should not be allowed to watch wrestling. I have seen kids use the moves they see in wrestling on one another. It wasn't a good sight to behold. I have seen a child pick up a kitchen knife and throw it at another child. Thank God it was the handle of the knife that struck the other kid's forehead. It would have been another story. He watched that move from an action movie and decided to try it out.

When I was much younger I saw a man putting a cigarette stick into his mouth, lighted it up and took a dip drag, then let the smoke out. When he was done smoking, he threw the cigarette butt on the floor.

The following day, as I saw it lying on the floor, I picked it up into the house, took a match stick and lit it up and began to do exactly what I saw the man doing the day before. I never knew what he was doing was wrong and unhealthy. I just copied him. That is how other kids copy ugly things too. That is why we as their parents must always watch over them.

Thank God I didn't end up smoking. It made no sense to me. I never got hooked on smoking. I never will.

A little kid was taken to the Juvenile delinquency for murder. He took out his dad's pistol and shot a boy his age. He did not know pulling the trigger would lead to the death of another child. He wanted to act on what he saw on television. His dad, who was a police officer, kept the gun in his drawer without locking it up.

He never in his wildest imagination would have thought that his son would attempt to pick up his loaded gun in his drawer and pull the trigger on his mate.

This is how children can be wasted via what they see in the media and in their immediate environment.

Parents caress themselves before their children. Some even go ahead to make love in the presence of their children saying, "What do they know? They are still little." These children can pick and practice these things when their parents are not at home.

Parents have returned home to see their children making love. They have committed incest. When they were asked how they came about what they were doing, they said they saw their parents doing it and decided to carry it out as an experiment.

A man who gives his toddler dry gin saying he wants his son to be strong is already opening the door of alcoholism into his son's life.

These and many more are what parents need to avoid so that they don't begin to regret their children. Parents are supposed to be happy with their children and not to weep over them. But when you do not do the needful, you may eventually be frustrated by them, later in life.

Let us do the needful now that we can correct and amend.

It's easier to train up a child than it is to repair an adult. The Lord will help us all.

The media is designed to take control over the minds of our children. The spirit of disobedience is at work in the lives of so many children in our generation.

Look at the below verses:

Proverbs 30:11 There is a generation that curseth their father, and does not bless their mother. Proverbs 30:12 There is a generation that are pure in their own eyes, and yet are not washed from their filthiness.

Proverbs 30:13 There is a generation, O how lofty are their eyes! and their eyelids are lifted up.

When you look at the above verses you will see that it falls in line with this present generation. Young boys have been badly influenced by social media. They hardly show respect to the elderly. They have no regard for anyone, not even their parents. They have been injected with the spirit of disobedience. The prince of the power of the air that the apostle Paul talked about in the book of Ephesians has succeeded in warping their minds and they are greatly influenced by these unclean spirits.

These kids smoke all kinds of deadly things and drink plenty of strong drinks. They get high and call it lifestyle but every responsible person knows they are wasting their lives.

These kids hardly listen to anyone. They are hard hearted and disobedient. If only their parents were there for them when they initially needed someone to direct them right. The sad reality is that these young stars would have destroyed their lives before someone would come to their rescue.

Our children need us. We must be there for them. If we are not, somebody else will. And that person may turn out to be a negative influence over them. When this happens in most cases, the influencer's voice over them tends to be louder than their parents' voice. This influencer's voice becomes the only voice they respect and obey. That is how powerful influence can be.

A child's life is centered around influences. If he receives positive influences, he will radiate positive energy. If he receives negative influences, he will in turn radiate negative energy.

Apart from influences from social media, we have peer group influences which could build positive behavior or mar the self esteem of young stars. The human mind has been programmed to learn new things every day. Our minds store information daily and this information can be good or bad. Positive information should be stored while negative information should be discarded.

However, the mind of a child is still developing and in most cases isn't mature enough to understand if an information is good for positive behavior or bad for negative behavior. A child just wants to copy whatever he or she sees, and hears.

Chapter 3

Train Up A Child

Proverbs 22:6 Train up a child in the way he should go: and when he is old, he will not depart from it.

Here in Nigeria, people respect families whose children are well behaved. No matter who you are, if your children are ill mannered, some certain kind of respect will be withdrawn from you.

God can't be lying when he says we should train up our children in the way they should go. In whatever way you want your child to go, you have the responsibility to commit them to training. If you take up the pain to train up your child in a godly way, he won't depart from that path of life.

A woman took her daughter to be delivered from the spirit of sexual immorality. When they stood before the prophet of God who was to deliver her, he said to the woman, "You are the architect of your daughter's misfortune. Your wealth is built on the foundation of prostitution. Your past life has robbed your daughter and that is why you see her doing the same thing you were doing in the past. Deliverance must first be conducted on you before we begin to set up a deliverance session for your daughter."

Training up a child takes a whole lot. It will take your time, effort, resources and even more. You cannot train your child in a hurry. You can't train them in impatience. Training up a child requires that you must be emotionally balanced. You also have to be mentally balanced, and physically balanced. You don't need all the money in this world to make a good behavior out of your child. Giving them love and tender care is better than buying them the whole world.

How do you train your child?

1. Train them in love.

Training up your child requires patience and patience can only be exhibited in love. You cannot train a child in hatred and resentment. You cannot train them in anger.

Children can be naughty , but a good spanking will give them common sense. But you have to be moderate in doing this. Do not over spank them so as not to begin to brood wickedness and hatred in them.

When you begin to over spank your child, he will develop a certain hatred for you. This attitude will make him see life differently and if this is not handled properly, it will spell doom in the near future.

I have heard children say, "I hate my dad. He flogs me all the time. He treats me rudely and harshly. He doesn't love me. The only thing he does is cane me. I am already used to being caned. I am no longer afraid when he canes me." When a child begins to act this way, he becomes more disobedient and stubborn and does what he pleases because he knows the only thing daddy will do is cane him.

It is not a good thing on the side of the man when everyone at home begins to run helter skelter at his arrival. You may feel they are all afraid of you which you presume it's a good thing but don't forget that pretense accompanies this kind of behavior.

Your children should run to you, jump on you, and hug you at your arrival. But when your entire household is as quiet as a graveyard because daddy is at home, and because everyone is scared, it means that you have lost connection with your family.

Your children are uncomfortable, sighing and unhappy because daddy is at home and the moment you are preparing to leave the house, there is jubilation, merriment, and excitement radiating all over them. This is a wrong way of training up your children. Please make necessary corrections and make your home a safe haven filled with joy, laughter, merriment, and harmony. Let's learn how to love not only our wives but our children too. Doing this will make them radiate in joy, and gladness at home and away.

There is a special joy that fills the heart of children when they see their parents. Ours should not be different. We must make them joyful the best way we can.

2. Prophesy Over Your Children

Too many parents are fond of using abusive words and curses on their children instead of pronouncing blessings on them.

The bible says in Proverbs 18:21, Death and life are in the power of the tongue: and they that love it shall eat the fruit thereof.

If there is indeed power in your tongue as the above bible verse implies, then you need to be extremely careful with the words you utter from your mouth. You must understand that only blessings should proceed from your mouth to your children and must from this moment desist at once from using abusive words and derogatory remarks on them.

In Genesis 49:3-7, we saw how Jacob, in anger, cursed his children, Reuben, Simon, and Levi and how those strong words reshaped their destinies.

In Genesis 2:19, the Bible says, "And out of the ground the LORD God formed every beast of the field, and every fowl of the air; and brought them unto Adam to see what he would call them: and whatsoever Adam called every living creature, that was the name thereof." Here is the scripture of emphasis,".. and whatsoever Adam called every living creature, that was the name thereof.

As a parent and a superior being over your children, you are the Adam in your family. Whatever you call your children is the exact thing they will become. You have the power to either speak good or evil over them. The power to build or break them lies in your tongue.

Satan understands this law quite frankly, so he moves you to always utter destructive words toward your children. He magnifies their weaknesses before you so that you will keep seeing their errors and insulting them in that way.

It is what Adam named them they become. In the same vein, it's what you name your children they will also become.

If you call them block-head, fool, idiot, stupid, cow, goat, and so on, that is what they will become. If you call them blessed, powerful, beautiful, handsome, bright, great and so on, they will become that also.

Parents may be wondering why their children perform badly in school or behave badly in public or act foolishly in important gatherings. It may be as a result of the words they have consistently been calling them. These words have robbed on them the character and behavior of a foolish, a idiotic, a stupid, and a block-headed child (ren). Reverse is also the case if you call them smart, intelligent, beautiful, loveable, and blessed children.

Any time I am to bathe my daughter, I will always decree positive words upon her and she always responds with an amen whenever those gracious words proceed from my mouth. I am building her destiny with those words because I have understood the power of the tongue as it relates to confessions and declarations.

Children are prone to mistakes and they can surely make one very upset. However, try not to allow their mistakes move you into an uncontrollable state of anger where you will begin to lay curses on them.

Don't utter words in anger. Learn to ignore the voices that move you to utter wrong words on them. First take a deep breath whenever you are annoyed and say nothing. It makes you feel better and the puff of anger can easily be deflated.

I have seen pregnant women curse their unborn child. They even curse their husbands whenever their labor pain intensifies. This is not good. You can convert the painful experience to prayer, ending every painful tear in your life, in the life of your husband and in the life of your baby. That's a better way to channel the pain in the right direction. Doing this will produce blessings and not curses.

You can begin today.

3. Pray Over Your Children

There is no better way to build up a child than in the place of prayer. You can't be with your children all day, but when you always pray over them, their guardian angels will always be on the lookout for them, executing the content of your prayer for their benefit.

Prayer can make your children walk in the right path of life. Ps. 32:8. Pro. 1:10.

Prayers can keep them from associating with bad and corrupt friends. Prayer can also keep them from strange children. Ps. 144:7.

Prayers can make your children walk in the absolute fear of the Lord. Don't forget to always mention their name in prayer. As a parent, you are their spiritual cover and they are under your spiritual radar.

It's not your pastor's sole responsibility to pray over your children but yours. So take that responsibility now. Your prayer is a spiritual searchlight that watches over them for safety and security.

With prayer you can secure the future of your children. It is what you say in the place of prayer that the angels assigned to them will carry out in their lives. Every prayer seed sown into their lives will definitely germinate and manifest at every appointed time in their lives. Keep building them in the place of prayer, at the end it will speak and you will always rejoice over them.

The prayer of Hannah made her first son Samuel a great prophet in Israel. 1Sam. 1:11.

The prayer of Abraham made Isaac a son of promise as spoken of by God. Gen. 25:5.

This is an eye opener for us all.

4. Give Your Children Sound Education

There is a song that goes thus, "Parents listen to your children. They are the children of tomorrow. Try to pay their school fee, and give them a sound education."

I lost my dad when I was very little. However, my mum took it upon herself by God's help to see that everyone of us were educated.

Imagine if my mum left us all uneducated, I wouldn't have been able to write this well for everyone to understand. I would not have been able to even publish these books for everyone to read.

Education is the bedrock of a nation. It's sad to know that a lot of parents don't cherish sound education. If your parents couldn't give you a sound education, don't transfer the aggression on your children. Do all you can to give them quality education to the best of your ability. When God sees your credibility in that area, he will send you help by either raising for you a financial pillar who will willingly sponsor their education or a scholarship board who will assist them get to the peak of their educational pursuit.

We are in a time where knowledge has greatly increased. And for anyone to be very impactful in this world, he or she needs adequate knowledge in his or her area of expertise.

Knowledge is not limited to place and time. The world has become a global village so you can learn about anything anywhere you are.

I am pleading with you parents not to use your children's tuition fees to buy clothes or shoes to look impressive. This may sound funny but it happens. I have experienced it.

I was teaching in a private primary school back then. There was this particular family who had three pupils in our school. They stopped coming to school for a while and I went in search of them only to discover that their mother used their school fees for a different purpose.

When their father discovered it, he told them to stay back until the matter was resolved. No father will be encouraged to pay for his children's tuition fee under such pretense by the mother. It's discouraging and heart breaking.

I am also pleading to fathers and mothers not to take their children's tuition fees to play sports betting. Always put their education first. This is very important.

Another thing I want to draw to your attention is the way and manner parents take their children out of school A and admit them in school B without settling the bills they are owing school A.

They have a little misunderstanding with either a teacher or head teacher in school A and without settling the dispute, they will literally take their children out of school A and admit them in school B. This kind of behavior is bad for your children.

Also be notified that if you must take away your children from school A to school B, make sure they are retained in the classes they were taken away from. Don't be too quick to put them in a higher class. Allow them to go through the process a step at a time.

Trying to put them in a higher class because you don't want to repeat paying tuition fees from the class they were taking may eventually have a negative effect on them. Remember that you are still trying to build up their mental strength and to achieve this, they must go through each process thoroughly.

We are to educate our children about?

1. Educate them about sex. It is a good thing to educate your kids about sex. It may sound weird but the earlier you educate them about sex the better. Do not say they are too small to learn about sex. Your educating them will equip them and keep them safe, making it difficult for them to be sexually molested. There are so many wild beasts out there putting on human skin. When it comes to sexual molestation, they don't have an age category or barrier.

They can sexually molest even a seven year old child. They are that beastly and animalistic. As your children grow up, it is advisable to take them deeper in the teaching of sex in line with genetic make-up as regards to changes in their physical structure. Let them know how to abstain from all kinds of sexual perversion including menstrual cycle if they are girls. If they get the lesson, they will hardly fall into sexual temptations that lead to sexually transmitted diseases, abortion, and unwanted pregnancies.

2. Educate them in their field of interest. Knowing the best educational program or module to give to your child(ren) is a great key that opens the door of achievement to them. There is no child without a gift or a talent. God has given each and every one of your children special abilities to be a contributor and a blessing to their world. If you notice that your child loves music, writing, singing or acting, then you should empower them with tools that can help them grow in their area. Whatever talent or gift they possess, help them to build it up and you will be glad you did. Don't be a source of discouragement to your children whenever they are trying to learn something new or trying to show you something they are interested in. You may not like what they are doing but please be patient with them, that may be their field of interest. And your discouraging words may make them lose interest which will later affect them in the future.

3. Educate them in your own fields of interest. No knowledge is wasted. The more educated your children are, the more successful they are likely to become. If you are a baker, kindly teach them how to bake during the holidays. You never can tell. That may be their source of living in the future. And if they are not interested in your field of interest please don't force them. Allow them to have a personal interest in your field of interest. When they do, growing in it will be easy, fun, and exciting.

4. Educate your child on the value of work. We live in a time where people cherish wealth more than work. They want to be wealthy

but they don't want to work. They look for the best possible way to get rich with little or no effort at all. They don't understand the value of work. If we must educate our children, we must educate them on the value of work. When we create an atmosphere of laziness around our children, they will grow up thinking that is the way life is. They won't want to put any effort into achieving anything in life. Parents who get their children enrolled in special centers to enable them pass their exams are doing great damage to their children. These kids will believe that they are ways to get things done without effort or work. Growing up with such a mindset is disastrous. You have gladly given them a wrong impression about the value of work. This will make them unable to make something meaningful out of life. And it will bring you shame and regrets in your latter life.

5. Educate them in the act of public speaking. Children who are not outspoken will be unable to stand up for themselves wherever they find themselves. Being bold and outspoken helps your child(ren) to stand their ground when confronted with a situation of peculiar interest. Children who are quiet and shy are looked down upon, ridden on, cheated, bullied, and taken for granted. But with an outspoken personality, the above set of unruly behaviors can't be exerted on them. Children who are timid and reserved suffer a lot in boarding schools. Such traits make them afraid of their tormentors. But those outspoken will be bold enough to report the case of their sufferings from bullies to the authorities which will in turn lead to the punishments of their offenders. You can begin to build up their confidence, boldness, self esteem, and level of outspokenness. Doing things will help them to become men and women who can stand for their rights and reclaim what belongs to them wherever they find themselves in life.

6. Educate your child(ren) about God. God is delighted when your child has reverence for him and godly fear. God is pleased when little children have a knowledge of who he is. Helping your

children to have a good relationship with Jesus is the best gift you can ever give to them. Teach your children how to pray at a tender age. Teach them how to read the bible. Teach them godly virtues and characters. Teach them how to please and love God. Teach and show them how to serve God with a good heart. Teach them the importance of serving God diligently and the importance of going to church early. Share testimonies of God's goodness to you and your family so they can learn to trust and depend solely on God in times of challenges. If you do this, you will be happy at the end. These teachings will empower them for life and they will in turn make you proud.

7. Educate your female children about indecent dressing. One of the easiest ways to sexually molest a female child is through indecent dressing. Your children are addressed the way they are dressed. Their dress sense can have a way of affecting the way people see, approach, and address them.

   As parents we can help our female children by carefully selecting the type of dresses they love to wear. When you go to the shopping mall to buy clothes, be careful to buy clothes that shuns indecency in every way. Don't allow the fashion trend of today's world to detect your children's dress sense. Clothes that are revealing spells doom especially to the girl child. If you ignore the signs and neglect the hand writing on the wall, you may have to be sorry when the unexpected happens. Don't let your girl child blame you tomorrow for the caution you neglected to take on their behalf today. Show them the dangers of indecent dressing and help them make right decisions. It's to your children's success.

One of the reasons God instituted marriage is for couples to raise godly children. Mal. 2:15. If that is properly understood, many parents will bring up their children in the way of the Lord.

When we fail to understand the purpose for making babies, we won't really care what exactly they do and how they tend to live their life as they grow up. But when we become fully aware that God gave us these children to be raised up in his own way, it becomes a delight to train them up in the way of the Lord.

Let us outline below some purposes for having children.

1. To have a godly heritage. Ps. 127:3. Our children are our heritage. They take after us when we are gone. Children are the posterity of parents. No matter how wealthy you are, if you have no child, you will have no choice but to transfer that wealth to either a charity organization, an orphanage, or even an NGO. Having a godly heritage is pleasing to the Lord. God does not want our serving him to end with us. He wants us to also teach our children his ways so that they can continue to serve him when we are gone. And he also wants our children to teach their children his ways so that they too can continue in servitude when they are gone. Serving God should not start and stop within one generation. It should continue from generation to generation. This is the desire of God.

2. To build up your spiritual defense. Ps. 127:4.

   Parents who have godly children have equipped themselves to resist spiritual forces and attacks. Godly children are arrows in the hands of their parents. They can be used to bring down an extremely dangerous enemy. When you raise godly children, you will have lesser burdens to bear because they can help you bear those burdens in the place of prayer. When your child is prayerful, it lessens the work. You won't be the only one raising a prayer altar while others are asleep. You are a blessed parent of your quiver full of godly children either biological or spiritual. Prayer will help them spring forth as arrows to their God ordained destinies.

3. To contend with the enemy. Ps. 127:5. Your children are your defense. You can't be put to shame when you are confronted with the battles that life brings. They will help you to contend, confront, and combat your enemies in the place of prayer. And by

the strength of God invested in them, they will fray the enemy and you will have peace on every side.

4. To imbibe godly virtues in them. One of the best things to leave your children with when you are gone are godly virtues. If you fail to do this, you will only labor in vain. Without godly virtues, your children will be a thorn in your flesh and you may end up cursing rather than blessing them. Without godly virtues, your children can destroy what you took years to build. But if you imbibe godly virtues in them, even if you did not leave any physical inheritance for them, they will greatly increase by the godly virtues embedded in them. Good books are the best gifts you can give to your children. You are not only molding their lives, you are also saving them from a lot of troubles. Get them a bible for them too and teach them how to read it. When you have done this, you have given them the best inheritance any parent can give to their children.

Chapter 4

The 5 As of Parenting

In this chapter, we shall be looking at five things parents can do to strengthen their relationship with their children.

1. Attention.

   Children are great attention seekers. They want you to listen to them when they talk and play with them when they come around you. Don't let them feel that you give more attention to your mobile phone and less attention to them. When your children realize that you pay more attention to other things than them, they will feel insecure around you. After all, you don't listen when they speak nor do you play with them when they run to you. They may be going through a problem that needs urgent attention and intervention but because their presence repels you, they will keep it to themselves and will have to face that challenge alone. And most times, they end up becoming a victim of the circumstances surrounding that challenge. When the damage has been done, you hear parents say to their children, "Why didn't you tell me, why didn't you come to me"? "You always shun me when I want to talk to you and tell me to go away when I want to play with you" are the kind of replies you will usually get in such cases as these. We can avoid such sad realities. We can turn a new leaf today and decide to keep our phones aside and pay more attention to the needs of our children.

   Your children may have all the physical needs of life but are very lonely and empty because mummy is too busy and daddy is never around. And they can get into the wrong hands while looking for a way to get rid of their state of loneliness and emptiness. When we place more priority on money than our children, our attention will be more on making money than tending to the emotional needs of our children. And such behaviors are capable of destroying the good relationship we should have with our children.

2. Affection

Showing love to your children is one of the best things you can do to them. Your love for your child has a great impact in his or her life. This even goes a long way to affect their adulthood. You cannot compare a child who was loved, cherished, and catered for to a child who was not. Your attitude towards your children has a strong influence on their minds. It tells if you love them or not.

A young girl was hated by her parents. The reason for the hatred was unknown. When she got fed up with the way she was being treated at home, she left the house and ran away to a friend's place. She afterwards got introduced to a gang of robbers. And when it was her turn to provide a target for their next operation, she suggested that her parents should be their next target. She told her gang members that she would love to be the one that would sparehead the operation so that she can pay her parents back for the evil they did to her during the course of her growing up with them. She saw their actions towards her as an act of wickedness and she was willing to make them cry because they will see her face to face. Their act of wickedness is what has turned her into a heartless being capable of doing great evil to anyone who falls prey.

When we see children become a menace to society when they become adults, it starts from their childhood. Everyone wants to be loved. When you transfer hate and aggression to your children, you are gradually producing in them corrupt seeds that will germinate into something destructive capable of damaging human lives. That is why a man will beat his wife, and a man would rape a little girl, and men will become terrorists, armed robbers, kidnappers, ritualists, cultists and so on. These ones were not loved. They were rather abandoned, forsaken, beaten, wounded, abused, cursed, and so on.

As a parent, please have it in mind that whatever seed you sow into your child will produce the same effect in greater quantity when it germinates. Let's try to show affection for our children. They will multiply the same in greater measure.

A young girl was raped by her mother's boyfriend when her mother wasn't around. She tried to explain to her mum what her boyfriend had done but she refused to believe her precious daughter and shunned her instead. This brought great damage to her emotions. She felt hated, abused, and abandoned. Years later she became a shadow of herself. She became a stripper and prostitute. She eventually went for a rehabilitation program to fight these demons and get her life back on track. On the final process of her program, she was on her way to submit the gun she acquired to kill her mother's boyfriend any day she sees him anywhere because he hurt her mother too and was on the run. She saw him that fateful day she was going to hand the gun over. The memories of her past life became so fresh again and with that anger, she pulled the trigger on him and he died on the spot. She was taken to prison and had to serve jail term. This became a terrible time for her. This is how neglecting a child can eventually become. The outcome is always devastating.

3. Accommodation

Apart from the fact that our children need our attention and affection, they also want us to accommodate them. As parents we may be very busy and may have a deadline to meet up a project or too busy with a contract or a term paper. We may be preparing for a message to be preached in church and therefore hide away from them or just want to be alone to think things through. As these are part of our everyday routine but we must also consider our children and their desire to be with us. We must try to get them room to encroach into our space. We must be able to accommodate them.

Accommodation helps our children to have a sense of belonging. They are part of our lives and must be attended to. They may more often than not want us to play with them at the wrong time but because we love them, we have to sometimes sacrifice that vital time and allow them to enjoy that moment they want to be with us. It's often difficult to do this but it's a vital role we must play. When we give our children that sense of belonging, we have succeeded in building their self esteem. They won't be afraid to come to us happily and cheerfully.

If you are an extremely busy parent, you can devise a way of creating time to accommodate your children. They need it to solidify their confidence, self esteem, and open mindedness towards you.

Some of us say it's tradition. That our children should not approach us anytime they want to because it could be termed as an act of disrespect. But if you understand how things work in the kingdom of God, you will allow God's word to overrule traditions of men and doctrines of devils.

God our father told us to approach him anytime, and anywhere. He said we should come boldly into his presence anytime. So if God who is sovereign can accommodate us without setting rules and regulations, then we must reciprocate the same to our children.

When a parent always resists his children from coming to his room, study, or his office, then he has something he is hiding. Let's give our children room into our lives now that we can and let's allow them to be free around us to help their sense of insecurity. The day is coming when you will wish your children are by your side because at that time, they have all gone their different ways and may also be too busy to attend to you the way you desire. Now is the time to have fun with your family. Spend quality time with them. Plant this good seed of accommodation in them. It will help them in life and in destiny. Be that awesome parent for your children. And when it's time for them to return the favor, you will definitely have nothing whatsoever to worry about.

4. Appreciation.

Everybody loves to be appreciated. How would your wife feel if after making your favorite meal, you just kept mute on her before and after eating? You didn't say a word of appreciation for the delicious delicacy she took time to cook and served you.

How would you feel if no one appreciates you after you work so hard to provide so much for your family? That same feeling is the way our children feel when we don't appreciate them, especially for a job well done. Children want to be appreciated especially when they attempt a seemingly impossible task. Why do you think your child kept talking about all the good things he did in your absence? He wants you to say something nice and encouraging to him. This makes him confident and proud of himself.

Have you ever noticed that children put more effort into their studies whenever they are promised a gift? They go that extra mile to make their parents glad when there is a gift attached to the task. To them, that gift is a symbol of appreciation and for this reason, they will make their parents very proud of them.

As parents we must not be too hard on our children. Some parents don't know how to appreciate their children. All they do is push them too hard and won't appreciate them for the little positive effort their children are putting in to make them proud. When you expect your child to finish top position in his class but he took third position, you should at least appreciate him and encourage him with a little gift. That child sincerely wants to take the top position. But he may have taken third due to some factors which weren't clearly his fault. This is where we as parents should stand by them and find out what would have transpired in the course of study or during the exams. We would definitely find the answer and help that child to come first next term. Whatever advancement our children are making, let us try to support, encourage and appreciate them for their strides. This will make them do more.

When we promise to appreciate our children when we want them to achieve the best in a task, we should play our own part by fulfilling our promise. Parents are fond of using this method to make their children achieve a feat but don't play their part when their children accomplish the task. This form of method is quite unhealthy. It may cause our children to lose their trust in us. They had believed with all their heart that we would fulfill our promise. So they went the extra mile to make us happy and when they expect their gift, we turn them down with excuses that are disappointing.

No one likes to be deceived. Not even us parents. Please let us render our all the promises due to them. Let us show them love and appreciate them when they make us proud. This is a call to parental duty.

5. Assistance.

As parents, it's our duty to assist our children in every way we can. Children love it when their parents assist them in their home work, and projects. When you assist your little child do his homework, you will be able to easily detect their shortcomings. You may notice they are pronouncing some letters or words wrongly and help them pronounce it right. You may also notice that they do not know how to write a particular alphabet or a number and as you notice it, you correct them.

Our teenage kids need our assistance in many areas. They need our help in getting educated about sex, menstrual cycle, peer group influence, physical body changes, and so on. They also need our assistance in making the right decision that will make their future great.

Discipline - A Better Approach to Child Upbringing.

When parents over pamper their children, they are not helping them in any way.

When parents allow the house help to do virtually all the house chores, they are not helping their children to receive proper home training. When we neglect giving our children the training they need when they are little, they will end up becoming a liability in the future.

In Nigeria, a lady who does not know how to cook is considered a liability. She would have problems with her husband if she eventually gets married. A typical Nigerian man loves eating healthy and homemade foods. He loves it more when it's being prepared by his wife. But if she doesn't know how to cook, it may bring discord in the home.

Whatever your children fail to learn or do when they are little would eventually be a thorn in their flesh when they become adults. If we fail to discipline our children when they are little and yield, it would be difficult to bend them when they are adults and can make certain decisions for themselves.

As parents, they are certain things we must not allow to happen in the life of our children.

A young man was sentenced to death by firing squad. When he was asked to mention his last wish, he asked that his mother should be brought to him. When she stepped up to him, he asked her to come closer and he wanted to tell her something in her ear. As she brought her ear close to his mouth, he bit her ear so badly that he tore out a part of the ear. She screamed in pain, holding her ear. Her hand was full of blood.

When he was asked why he treated his mother in such an unkind way, he told a story of how his mother became the architect of the legacy he has built. She never cautioned him about all he did wrong. She never questioned him whenever he brought another pupil's things home. She defended him any time his dad tried to interrogate him. By this he grew up becoming an armed robber. When he brings goodies home, she never bothered to ask how they came about. She just cheers him and encourages him in her ignorance. He lost his life and his mother lost part of her ear. If she had disciplined her child when he was little, she would have been joyous in the future. It's what you sow you shall reap.

Steps To Proper Discipline

1. Put an eye on your children

   As a parent, observation is very paramount. You must observe the behavior of your children and spot the changes in their character makeup. If any of your child begins to act indifferent, you must checkmate him or her to find out what exactly may be the problem for the new type of behavior he or she is putting up. When an outspoken child becomes withdrawn, something is definitely wrong. You must as a parent treat whatever has caused that withdrawal urgently. You mustn't assume or conclude in your mind what you may think may be the cause of such behavior. You must ask your child and be intentional to find out what exactly may be the problem. He or she will open up to you. And if they may not want to tell, please don't quit. Keep pushing until you get to the bottom of it. It will save you a lot of trouble.

   Many children are going through hell. Their parents may be too busy with work, business, and traveling. They are not around for their children and are no more sensitive to their children's emotional needs. You may be a very hard working parent and you are doing a great job of providing all for your children's physical needs. However, there are other needs to be met like mental and emotional needs. These needs are only met when parents are always around for their kids. The current economic state of things may be a major reason many parents don't have time for their children but we must strike that balance between work and family if we must save our children and build a solid foundation for our home.

A child doesn't just become a cultist overnight. Negligence to parental duties is a major factor to this. When you are always too far away from your kids, you can't tell who their friends are, who they relate with on a daily basis, who they hang out with on weekends and their whereabouts, it will be difficult to correct, reprove, and instruct them. Many parents have cried bitterly over their children when they discovered what they have eventually become. You can imagine being called from school or from the police station or from any other unlikely places that you should immediately report for an urgent matter which has to do with the involvement of your child in an unspeakable act. That alone can have adverse effects on your health.

The act of discipline is an act of firmness. You can't afford to lose your sanity because of your child whom you consider irritating or obstinate. A good caning can go a long way to helping him adjust to the pattern or choice of behavior you attended to imbibe in him. When a child is lazy, a good spanking can cause him to change. An unruly child can be cultured. Those bad behaviors can be curtailed by some good spanking.

Proverbs 23:13 Withhold not correction from the child: for if thou beatest him with the rod, he shall not die. 23:14 Thou shalt beat him with the rod, and shalt deliver his soul from hell.

Those lashes with a cane you are giving your children will save them from danger. It will deliver them from destruction. Please make good use of the cane. Be intentional and with discretion. It's a life saver.

Another thing a parent must observe is what their children bring home. Ask valid questions when your child brings whatever does not belong to him or her home. Get the actual facts behind what he or she is in possession of.

If you feel you are being kept in the dark by your child and you have a feeling that he is just being silent over an issue you think he should talk about. You can find a way to let him speak up. You can go further to quietly search his room or his school bag for any information you need to enable you to solve the mystery he refused to unravel.

Another important way of keeping an eye on your children is by paying them unannounced visits in school. You will be able to observe real life situations. Especially if they are in boarding school, college of Education, polytechnic or in the university. Taking this step may help you address areas like his set of friends, mode of dressing, level of seriousness in his studies and so on.

2. Limit their level of exposure to social media

Another way to discipline your children is to limit their level of exposure to social media. It is true that we are in the era of information technology and there are a lot of things our children can gain from the internet. However, too much exposure will lead them astray. The internet is full of all kinds of things and the social media of this age tries to put all kinds of immoral things in your face. Through this channel, a lot of children have been trapped. They keep late nights watching movies, engaging in online dating sites, and exploring sites that are not moral for young minds. Some even go deeper into learning how to play sports betting, gambling, and committing cyber fraud. With the internet, the world is not at our fingertips and if we don't limit our children to the level of exposure they can get from the web, it will mess up their innocent minds, distort their vision and corrupt their values. It's important to set a limit because the internet has no age restrictions. It has no parental guidance. It's just free to air and open for all to explore.

3. Help them to have passion for books

> Reading is one thing that can help anyone attain success. Children prefer playing to studying. They infer that studying is boring but playing is fun. Children don't want to be disturbed. They prefer to eat, play, and sleep. They just want to remain in that state of pleasure. But if we want the best for our children, we mustn't just put them in a good school but teach them how to love reading.

> Get books that are catchy and colorful to the eyes. Books with illustrations and drawings are very fun to read. Learning could be fun. Children love to have fun so if you get them books that make learning fun, they will love reading. The moment they imbibe that good reading habit, it becomes easy to read even when they are all by themselves. With this habit of reading and studying, their future is bright and they can become anything they want to be.

Words For Men

Dear fathers, as the head of the family, we have the responsibility of taking good care of our family. We must also learn to assist our wives in every little way we can. Our wives need us to take care of things at home. Men love sex. It's only when your wife isn't stressed she can comply with your demand for sex. She doesn't have to be the only one doing the dishes, changing the diaper, bathing the baby, cooking the meals, doing the laundry, cleaning and sweeping. We as husbands have to assist our wives in the aforementioned areas too. Have you ever tried doing the things your wife does at home everyday, it really works and could be very demanding. If we help them in some of these chores, they will be restful, healthy, and energetic. A lot of women are already in a mess. They look so stressed and weak due to excessive home chores. Nobody is helping out. And after all that tiredness, the husband still comes to demand for sex. And when she tries to explain why she won't be able to give him, he flares up, and says all kinds of derogatory words to his wife.

This isn't ought to be so. We can always enjoy our wives' company. All it requires is a little helping hand. Let's imbibe this into our families.

As fathers, our children see us as their role model. We have to be there for them. We have to love them, teach them and show them the importance of our values, our beliefs, and our legacy.

Our children should be able to look upon us as fathers and be proud to call us their fathers. They should be glad to call us daddy and be grateful to God for making us their fathers. We should not become an object of public ridicule and make our children and family ashamed because of us. Our children deserve the best from us. Let's give them our best and they will continue to pray for us.

Words For Women

Dear mothers, I understand the magnitude of work you have put into the upbringing of your children. You conceived them in your womb and brought them forth into this world. I know the pain you go through and the effort you put in for your children to have a better life. And God will indeed reward your labor of love towards your lovely children.

In addition to this, please mothers, don't be the instrument of destruction in your home. You have the power to build the home. You spend more hours with the children than we men. So their growing up lies more in your effort. As mothers, please don't begin to compare your children to that of your neighbor or what have you. You must unite your home and make your family stand out. Also, love your children equally. Don't make unhealthy comparisons among your children. God has created them uniquely.

Moreso, pray fervently for your home and children. Also stand by your husband in every way you can. He needs you to overcome all the hurdles that will come at him from time to time.

Make the home a peaceful and safe place to live. Your home must never be a wrestling ring. You have the power to make your home a safe haven.

May God bless you and help you and your husband to accomplish this in every way possible in Jesus' mighty name.

I love you with the love of the Lord.

ABOUT FRANCIS .A. UWANDU

Born in 1984 in Lagos State Nigeria, Francis Uwandu grew up without adequate nurturing by his father. He died at a young age. Left alone to take care of her five beloved children, his mother worked so hard in order for Francis and his siblings to continue their education.

He eventually became a graduate with a degree in Psychology, University of Ibadan in 2010. Those formative years in the University was where he discovered God and realized he had a calling. It was in these formative years he discovered he could write books.

Via his writings, he has been able to touch multitudes near and far.

Other books written by the same author are; The Blood Book, Motiv-8 (8 Practical Steps To Enhance Motivation, The Blood Speaks, Why Christians Go To Hell, The Living Meal and many yet unpublished manuscripts.

www.ingramcontent.com/pod-product-compliance
Lightning Source LLC
Chambersburg PA
CBHW071016260726
48661CB00007B/3001